D0444843

Rheumatoid Arthritis

Decrease or reverse symptoms–naturally

alive books

Vancouver
Canada

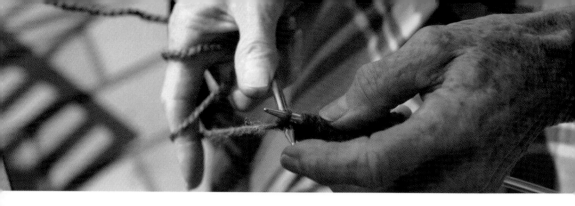

C o n t e n t s

Note: Conversions in this book (from imperial to metric) are not exact. They have been rounded to the nearest measurement for convenience. Exact measurements are given in imperial. The recipes in this book are by no means to be taken as therapeutic. They simply promote the philosophy of both the author and *alive* books in relation to whole foods, health and nutrition, while incorporating the practical advice given by the author in the first section of the book.

Recipes

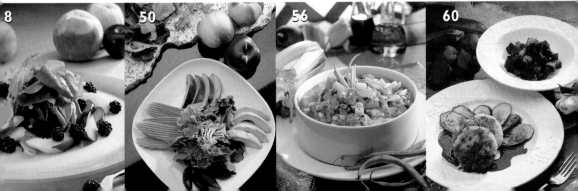

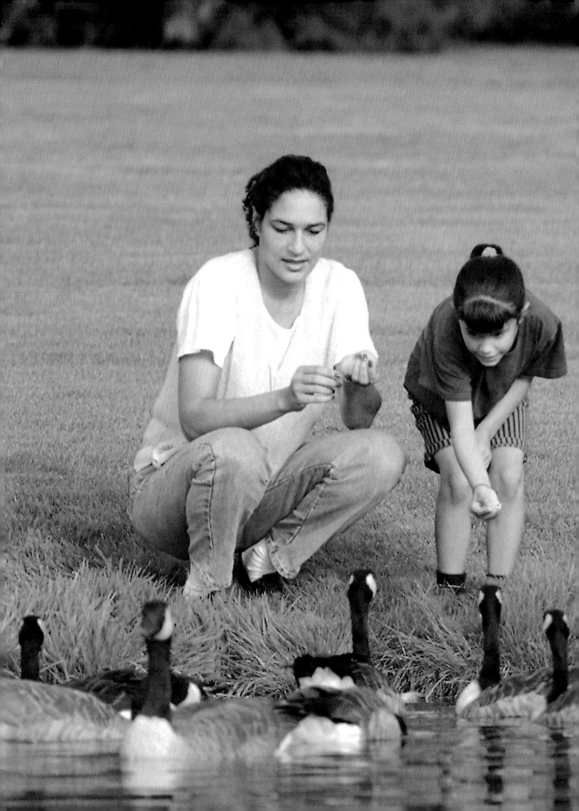

Conventional medical authorities claim that there is no cure for rheumatoid arthritis. Drug use may provide pain relief; however, it does little, if anything, to alter the arthritic process itself.

Introduction . . . .

When we hear the term "arthritis," we usually think of cracking joints and stiffness in the morning. This vision is an accurate one; however, rheumatoid arthritis is a more destructive form of arthritis than the well-known *osteo*arthritis that affects most seniors. The inflammation associated with rheumatoid arthritis can cause crippling and deformation of joints at an early age. In fact, rheumatoid arthritis can affect anyone, including children.

Rheumatoid arthritis is an autoimmune disease, which means that the body attacks its own tissues as a result of faulty immune system reaction. The true cause of this condition is unknown. That's why it's so important to try to understand what triggers inflammatory attacks, and what worsens or triggers symptoms.

Conventional authorities claim that there is no cure for rheumatoid arthritis. The primary treatment of rheumatoid arthritis is with various medications, which, like in the case of non-steroidal anti-inflammatory drugs, actually accelerate the destructive nature of the disease.

The natural approach to rheumatoid arthritis, however, goes beyond mere management or masking of symptoms to address the underlying systemic problems. Rheumatoid arthritis *can* be reversed, provided that the joints and affected organs are not irreversibly damaged .

Medical authorities claim there is no cure for rheumatoid arthritis.

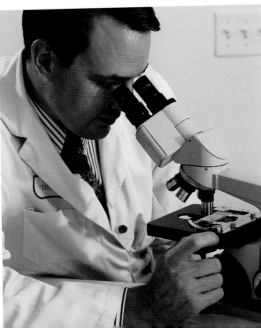

Sandy Wright

There are a number of natural approaches to decreasing the symptoms of, or reversing, rheumatoid arthritis. Following a hypoallergenic diet (a diet free from food allergies), for example, will bring the most dramatic benefits to those suffering from this condition. There are many supplements and alternative therapies that help people live with or eliminate this condition. The only sure way to either cure or deal with rheumatoid arthritis successfully is to educate yourself.

What is Rheumatoid Arthritis? . . . .

Rheumatoid arthritis (RA) is a systemic disease of altered immunity–an autoimmune disease–affecting not only the joints but also the eyes, muscles, nerves and other organs. People suffering with it often feel exhausted and ill, and may have anemia and chronic muscle pain in addition to the joint disease.

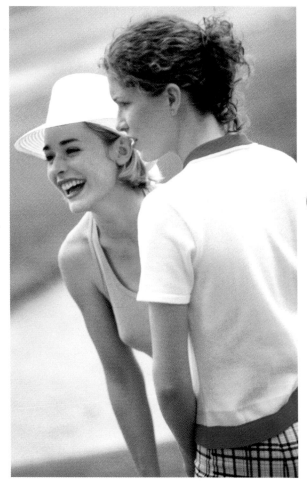

While this condition is most commonly developed in people between the ages of twenty-five and fifty (women are affected three times more than men), it can occur at any age. About 3 percent of the population (an estimated three million North Americans) suffers from rheumatoid arthritis.

Rheumatoid arthritis is one of those diseases that waxes and wanes, with occasional remissions lasting weeks, months and even years. Rheumatoid arthritis does reduce the average life expectancy by three to seven years due to complications such as infection, gastrointestinal bleeding and other side effects caused by drugs taken for the condition.

Women are affected by rheumatoid arthritis three times more than men.

The Start and Spread of Rheumatoid Arthritis . .

Rheumatoid arthritis usually starts slowly over a number of months or years. Symptoms include fatigue, loss of appetite, weakness and vague muscle aches and pains. There may not be any joint pain but at some point joint pain appears, with warmth, swelling, tenderness and stiffness after inactivity of the joint.

Rheumatoid arthritis usually affects only a few joints initially but slowly progresses to many other joints. The joints most frequently affected are the hands, wrists, elbows, shoulders, knees and ankles. In some cases the hips, jaw and neck joints may also be affected.

The inflammatory process of RA first affects the synovium, the membrane that surrounds a joint and creates a protective sac. This sac is filled with lubricating liquid–the synovial fluid. This fluid cushions the joint and supplies nutrients and oxygen to cartilage, a slippery tissue that coats the ends of bones. When the synovium becomes inflamed it secretes more fluid. Later, the cartilage becomes inflamed and damaged. The cartilage and supporting structures around the joint are eventually destroyed and cause the characteristic RA deformities.

The joints most frequently affected by rheumatoid arthritis are the hands, wrists, elbows, shoulders, knees and ankles.

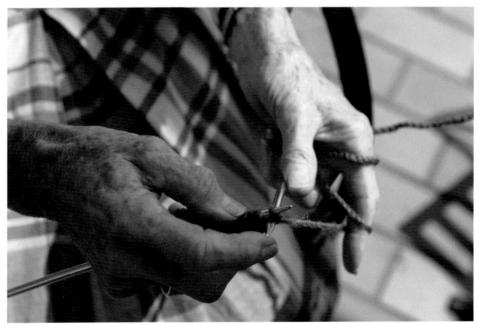

Cartilage

Cartilage is basically made up of a protein called collagen. Collagen forms a mesh to give support and flexibility to joints. With RA there is a continuous inflammation of the synovium and a gradual destruction of the collagen, which causes a narrowing of the joint space and eventually damage to the bone.

In progressive RA the fluid and inflammatory cells accumulate in the synovium to produce a pannus–a growth composed of thickened synovial tissue. The pannus produces more enzymes that destroy nearby cartilage, aggravating the area and attracting more inflammatory white cells, leading to more inflammation. This inflammatory process can also affect organs in other parts of the body.

What Causes Rheumatoid Arthritis?

Rheumatoid arthritis is initiated by a process called autoimmunity, in which the body's white blood cells (T-cells) mistake the body's own collagen cells as foreign antigens (allergens) and set off a series of events to rid the body of the perceived threat. Other white blood cells (lymphocytes) called B-cells then produce antibodies (auto-antibodies) that attack the body's synovium. The cause of this autoimmunity is controversial. Some say it is due to a genetic susceptibility.

Others say an infection with a virus may be involved as the triggering event.

Still others claim bacteria, parasites, fungi or chemicals of different kinds may be the triggering factors.

Severe stress such as that experienced with the death of a family member,

Triggers for the onset of rheumatoid arthritis include severe stress and significant injury.

Sandy Wright

9

a divorce or separation, loss of a job, or a significant injury can all trigger the onset of RA.

Over the years, several patients of mine who had been free of arthritis developed the condition shortly after a car accident produced a whiplash neck injury. And rheumatoid arthritis seems to be occurring more and more often in people suffering from fibromyalgia, the subject of one of my other books in this series (*Fighting Fibromyalgia, alive* Natural Health Guides #20, 2000). Cold, wet weather can also trigger RA in some genetically predisposed individuals. Approximately two-thirds of people with RA begin their disease in the winter when infections are more common.

Whatever the trigger, the mechanism of inflammatory damage is the same. White blood cells stimulate the production of two proinflammatory chemicals called leukotrienes and prostaglandins. The leukotrienes attract even more white blood cells to the area while the prostaglandins open blood vessels and increase blood flow.

It is important to know that the body also produces anti-inflammatory prostaglandins that can offset the proinflammatory kind and produce symptom relief.

White blood cells also produce cytokines, small proteins that cause joint damage and may even be responsible for inflammation that occurs in parts of the body beyond the joints. Cytokines in small amounts are indispensable for healing. However, if overproduced they can cause serious damage including fever, shock and liver damage.

Signs and Symptoms of Rheumatoid Arthritis

Rheumatoid arthritis manifests itself with several characteristic signs and symptoms. It generally begins as morning stiffness and pain in the small joints of the hands and the feet, progressing to involvement of the larger joints and the joints of the cervical (neck) spine.

Since it is a systemic disease–involving the whole system–many other major signs and symptoms other than that of the joints will be seen.

The major signs and symptoms are:
- Fatigue
- General discomfort, uneasiness or ill feeling (malaise)
- Loss of appetite
- Low-grade fever
- Joint pain, joint stiffness and joint swelling (usually symmetrical; may involve the wrist, knee, elbow, finger, toe, ankle or neck)
- Limited range of motion
- Morning stiffness
- Deformities of hands and feet
- Round, painless nodules under the skin

Other signs and symptoms are:
- Skin redness or inflammation
- Patchy skin color
- Paleness
- Mouth sores
- Swollen glands
- Eye burning, itching and discharge
- Ear noise/buzzing

Rheumatoid arthritis is characterized, in about 25 percent of cases, by what are called rheumatoid nodules. These are painless, hard round or oval masses (aggregations of cells) that appear under the skin, usually on pressure points such as the elbow, wrist or Achilles tendon. They can also appear in the eye, causing inflammation, as well as in the lungs, leading to inflammation of the lining of the lung (pleurisy) and shortness of breath.

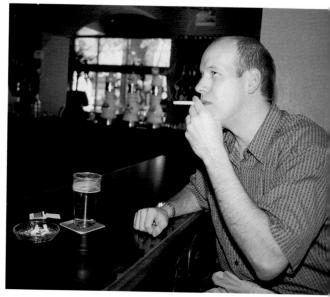

Lifestyle factors are significant in the development of rheumatoid arthritis.

Anemia may also occur with RA due to failure of the bone marrow to produce enough new red cells, but iron supplements will not help this anemia. The anemia is actually caused by the disease process itself, which affects the bone marrow. In order to treat the anemia, one has to be able to first control the disease itself. Other problems encountered with RA are muscle weakness and atrophy. In some cases the heart muscle becomes weakened and congestive heart failure may result.

Rheumatoid vasculitis (inflammation of the blood vessels) is yet another serious complication of RA that can be life threatening because it can lead to skin ulcerations, bleeding intestinal ulcers and diseases of the nervous system. Vasculitis can also cause skin rashes, Raynaud's phenomenon and massive hemorrhage from the gut.

12

There are many criteria for diagnosing rheumatoid arthritis.

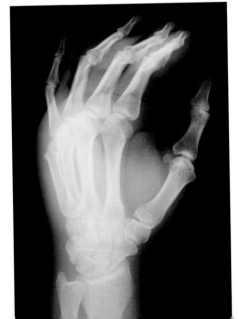

Diagnosing Rheumatoid Arthritis . . . .

People often ask me how a doctor knows whether a person has rheumatoid arthritis. There are several objective tests that can help make the diagnosis. First, since over 70 percent of patients with RA have a high level of an antibody in their blood called rheumatoid factor (RF), a positive RF blood test is one way of diagnosing the disease. Unfortunately, the RF level could also be elevated in the presence of many other diseases, including systemic lupus erythematosus and chronic liver disease. If RF values (also called titers) are very high, this tends to be associated with more severe forms of RA and is a poor prognosis.

The American College of Rheumatology lists the following additional diagnostic criteria that go along with the RF test:
- X-ray evidence of joint erosion
- Symmetrical arthritis
- Morning stiffness lasting at least an hour
- Arthritis of the hand joints
- Arthritis affecting three or more joint areas
- The presence of rheumatoid nodules

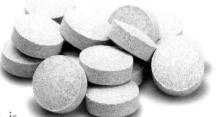

In about 90 percent of cases, a blood test called the erythrocyte sedimentation rate (ESR) is elevated. About 80 percent will have what is termed an "anemia of chronic disease" (normocytic-normochromic anemia). Another frequently abnormal blood test finding in RF is an elevated plasma fibrinogen level.

The drugs prescribed for rheumatoid arthritis may offer temporary pain relief; however, they do nothing to improve the condition and cause seriously harmful side effects.

Conventional Medical Treatment . . . .

Conventional medical authorities claim that there is no cure for rheumatoid arthritis. The primary treatment of RA is with various medications such as ASA and nonsteroidal anti-inflammatory drugs (NSAIDS). These drugs may offer temporary pain relief but they are accompanied by side effects such as gastrointestinal ulcers and bleeding.

Nonsteroidal anti-inflammatory drugs are the most common therapy for arthritis, and they are big business for the pharmaceutical companies. Unfortunately, they cause bleeding from the gastrointestinal tract in close to 25,000 people a year in North America. What's more, there is now evidence that these drugs accelerate the destructive nature of the disease.

Although drug use may provide pain relief, it does little, if anything, to alter the arthritic process itself. The natural approach to rheumatoid arthritis, however, goes beyond mere management of symptoms to address the underlying systemic problems that are associated with the condition. And provided that the joints and affected organs are not irreversibly damaged, rheumatoid arthritis can be reversed. First and foremost it is necessary to understand and ameliorate the leaky gut syndrome phenomenon. The leaky gut syndrome is at the root of practically all autoimmune diseases (see page 28).

A new class of NSAIDS called Cox-2 inhibitors (e.g., Celebrex®, Vioxx®) have recently been put on the market and, so far, appear to have fewer side effects than ibuprofen, fenoprofen and others, especially with respect to gastrointestinal bleeding problems. Doctors seem to be prescribing these drugs with a passion, but the long-term consequences of their use are, at this writing, unknown.

Corticosteroids (e.g., Prednisone) are sometimes used to reduce inflammation but their use is limited to short-term courses because of potential side effects. Side effects may include bruising, thinning of the bones (osteoporosis), hip fractures, cataracts, weight gain, susceptibility to infections, diabetes and high blood pressure.

Some doctors use gold compounds, chelation drugs, anti-malarial medications, and anti-cancer drugs (chemotherapy) as treatment modalities. Immunosuppressive drugs (similar to chemotherapy) are also used for people in whom other therapies have failed. All these medications may be used for weeks or months and are associated with toxic side effects like bone marrow, liver and kidney failure.

Other conventional RA treatments are physical therapy (to increase range of motion) and surgery aimed at relieving the signs and symptoms of the disease. Surgery can sometimes relieve joint pain, correct deformities and modestly improve joint function.

Natural Treatment for Rheumatoid Arthritis ..

Over the past 20 years I have developed an effective natural treatment protocol for reducing the level of symptoms as well as, in some cases, reversing the disease process of rheumatoid arthritis. Most of this protocol can be done in conjunction with conventional treatments; however, effectiveness is enhanced if drugs are not also used. The protocol is best done with the help of a natural health care provider, although it can be undertaken with a high degree of safety without practitioner input.

I have listed the various components of the natural treatment protocol in order of greatest to least importance. My experience tells me that the results are best when all steps are followed.

You will still see improvement or benefit even if you only use a few of the treatment protocol recommendations. Everyone is different so it is difficult to say which step will work best for you. My advice is to try to find a health care provider to work with. If none is available close to where you live, follow these steps as best you can.

The worst that can happen is nothing. At best, you may be able to reverse your disease or put it into remission for years to come.

Food Allergies

The single most effective natural treatment for rheumatoid arthritis, and the one that will result in the most dramatic benefits, is to follow a hypoallergenic (free of food allergies) diet. The signs and symptoms of all autoimmune disorders, including rheumatoid arthritis, can be either reversed or significantly reduced in severity with the detection and elimination of allergic foods and chemicals.

While these allergies are not necessarily the cause of the autoimmune condition, they most certainly can trigger flare-ups of symptoms or exacerbate existing symptoms such as morning stiffness, joint and muscle pain, fatigue and all manner of digestive upsets.

Undetected food allergies are extremely common and can be the root cause of morning stiffness and joint pain. There are two kinds of adverse reactions to foods: delayed and immediate. Wheezing, hives and swelling are examples of immediate reactions, occurring moments to a few hours after consuming the offending food. These kinds of reactions, however, comprise only 10 percent of all food allergies. The vast majority occurs on a delayed basis, up to four days later.

Fresh organic fruits, provided you are not allergic to them, are a part of a healthful whole foods diet.

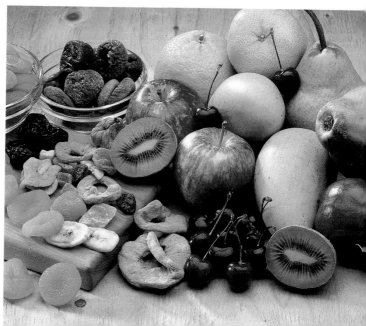

Food Allergies: Immediate and Delayed Reactions

To understand which types of tests are valid and reliable in determining food and chemical allergies, it is important to realize that there are basically only two kinds of adverse reactions: delayed and immediate.

Immediate Reactions

- allergic symptoms (e.g., wheezing, swelling, choking, pain) commonly occur two hours or less after consumption of the offending foods or chemicals; the food or chemical reaction is usually well known to the subject
- only one or two foods are involved in causing allergic signs and symptoms, which are usually severe; for example, the well-known and often life-threatening reactions to peanuts, shellfish and strawberries
- food or chemical reactions are triggered by even trace amounts of foods; it may take only the odor of cooked lobster to elicit intense allergic reactions in sensitive individuals
- common in children and rare in adults
- usually a permanent or "fixed" allergy; these food reactions can be lessened by vitamin, mineral and herb supplementation
- associated with the IgE family of antibodies, and can be verified by a skin test or a blood test called the IgE RAST (Radio-Allergo-Sorbent-Tests)

Delayed Reactions

- allergic reactions usually occur within twenty-four hours but sometimes up to four days after consumption of the offending foods or chemicals
- anywhere from three to twenty foods may be involved in causing allergic signs and symptoms, which are usually chronic (joint and muscle pain, fatigue, depression, psoriasis, etc.) and are hidden or unsuspected by the victim
- food or chemical reactions occur after consuming large amounts of foods, often in multiple feedings; a single food challenge might not cause any allergic reactions to occur
- very common in children and adults; there are over fifty medical conditions and 200 symptoms triggered, worsened or caused by the allergic reactions
- usually reversible within three to six months with a combination of food elimination and nutritional supplement therapy (antioxidants, enzymes, herbs, etc.)
- can be verified by blood tests known as the ELISA/Act test, the non-IgE RAST and the FICA (Food Immune Complex Assay)

Most authorities agree that the elimination-provocation technique is the most accurate way to detect food allergies. This involves following a hypoallergenic diet for three weeks, eliminating the most common food allergens: wheat, corn, dairy, citrus, eggs, chocolate. Thereafter, the body is challenged with the eliminated foods one by one, and reactions are noted.

During the elimination diet, most people's symptoms improve (stiffness, joint pain, etc.). If symptoms return when a food is reintroduced, you're probably allergic to that food.

Allergy Lab Tests

One can also identify hidden food allergies using skin tests or blood tests (e.g., the ELISA/Act or IgG RAST blood test). The drawback to skin testing is that it's designed to detect immediate reactions to foods. Since over 90 percent of food allergies are of the delayed onset type, skin tests cannot identify the vast majority of food allergies. Blood tests measure antibodies in the blood directed at specific foods. Results can be misleading, however, if you're taking cortisone, acetylsalicylic acid, antihistamines or other drugs.

To do this test, all that's needed is a single drop of blood. Food allergy home testing kits allow you to test for up to 100 foods through a drop of blood taken from the fingertip. You can obtain this in the privacy of your home without consulting a doctor.

York Laboratories in England accepts such blood samples from all over the world. The lab then processes the blood to determine the level of antibodies against specific foods. Positive test results are close to 100 percent accurate but there may be false negatives, in that the test may miss up to 20 percent of allergies. (See the appendix for further information.)

If you can neither afford testing through a lab like York or a natural health care provider, the elimination-provocation test may be your only diagnostic option. Having said this, I must also acknowledge the fact that many people who are in agony with crippling arthritis find it difficult to impossible to stick to an elimination diet for any length of time. The good news, however, is that close to 100 percent of RA victims will benefit by simply following a basic hypoallergenic diet.

The vast majority of cases of RA tested for food allergies show antibodies to gluten (from wheat) and/or casein (dairy protein), and benefit from a diet that eliminates dairy and all grains except rice, all refined carbohydrates, caffeine, red meats and processed foods. The majority of rheumatoid arthritis victims will also do better if they give up caffeine, alcohol and other stimulants, as well as "excitotoxins" like monosodium glutamate, aspartame and hydrolyzed protein. Alcohol should definitely be avoided because of its tendency to impair liver detoxification pathways that clear toxins emanating from inflamed joints. Carbonated beverages high in phosphates should also be eliminated since they can deplete calcium and magnesium from the body, two minerals RA victims are usually deficient in. Deficiency of calcium and magnesium worsens joint pain and stiffness.

The Inflammatory Response

It has been known for eons that water or juice fasting for periods of several weeks either greatly improves or reverses rheumatoid

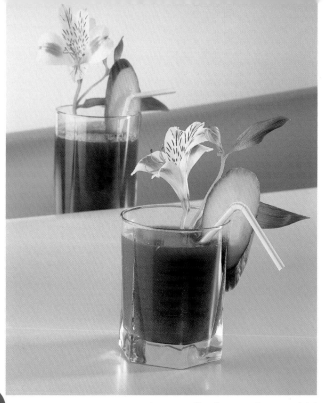

arthritis. The reason fasting can be so beneficial is that it reduces or eliminates the levels of circulating antibodies and "antigen-antibody complexes" created by food allergies.

Antibodies are made by our white blood cells in response to an antigen—a substance that is perceived by the immune system as an invader needing to be neutralized. An antigen-antibody complex is formed, and this elicits an inflammatory response. When the immune system reacts aggressively to a food, the antigen-antibody reaction could lead to a chronic inflammatory state every time you consume that "allergic" food. Knowing what foods to eliminate reduces inflammation and subsequent disease.

Water or juice fasting for several weeks greatly improves or reverses rheumatoid arthritis.

Most people with food allergies are unaware of their condition because in a delayed reaction the symptoms may occur many hours or days after ingestion. Delayed food allergies often create a complex blend of symptom-masking effects, withdrawal reactions and symptom reproduction with food reintroduction. Those with food allergies can behave as if they were addicted to foods. People often crave the foods that cause their symptoms and this is one fairly reliable way of knowing what should be taken out of their diets to improve their immune status.

Sorting Out the Confusion

Since over 90 percent of all food allergies are of the delayed onset type, skin tests and the IgE RAST will miss detecting the vast majority of food allergies. Nevertheless, conventional doctors continue to use them for that purpose, and often conclude that the patient does not have any food allergies even though no tests were ever done for delayed hypersensitivity food reactions. For this and other reasons, those suffering from arthritis, asthma, chronic sinusitis, hay fever, recurrent respiratory tract infections and other diseases are told that food allergies have nothing to do with their illness and that only a lifetime of steroid, antibiotic and antihistamine drugs will help.

There are many good tests that help detect food and chemical reactions. Although considerable confusion exists about which laboratory test is best, most agree with the accuracy and reliability of the elimination-provocation technique described by food allergy pioneers such as Drs. William Crook and Doris Rapp. This technique involves eliminating whole classes of foods for several days, then adding them back and noting reactions. Workable variations of this are the Coca Pulse Test and sublingual food tests. Some of these procedures would not be appropriate for those who do not have the time or stamina to experiment with their diets, or for people suffering from severe pain syndromes. On the other hand, there is something to be said for experiencing the effects of allergenic foods in reproducing symptoms. The elimination-provocation technique ultimately empowers sufferers to control symptoms with simple diet changes.

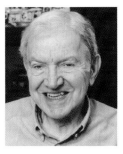

Dr. William Crook was one of the food allergy pioneers to advocate the elimination-provocation technique.

The Elimination-Provocation Test

The basic concept behind this type of food allergy testing is to follow a hypoallergenic diet for three weeks, eliminating the most common food allergens and thereafter challenging the body with the eliminated foods one by one, noting the reactions. During the three-week elimination diet, symptoms improve in the majority of people who suffer from food allergies.

If the reintroduction of certain foods causes a reproduction of the symptoms, the person is probably allergic to those foods. This diet works only if all the foods to be discontinued are done so abruptly or "cold turkey." Easing into this diet slowly or with some other compromise does not work nearly as well. In severely ill people (cancer, heart disease, diabetics, cortisone-dependent asthmatics or other life-threatening problems), it is not recommended that this approach be tried without close supervision by a medical doctor. Use common sense and the advice of your naturopath or doctor before attempting this on your own.

The elimination-provocation test (when appropriate) combined with the ELISA/Act test is currently state-of-the-art in detecting hidden food allergies. The scientific literature certainly supports this approach. The advantage of the ELISA/Act test is that it is capable of detecting delayed food allergies.

This in no way invalidates other forms of testing that may work equally well for selected people. In the future, with more research, time and practitioner experience, the question of test validity and reliability will become clearer. In the meanwhile, people who eliminate the offending foods from their diets reduce the allergic load on the immune system. This gives the body the opportunity to repair damaged tissues like the joints, muscles or the lining of the respiratory tract. Those who are allergic to dust, ragweed, pollens and other inhalant allergies can then be more tolerant to environmental allergens and less likely to suffer from severe allergic reactions that previously needed strong drugs for control.

The Rheumatoid Arthritis Diet . . . .

The following recommendations are general guidelines only and should be modified depending on individual food tolerances or allergies. Nightshades foods (tomatoes, potatoes, peppers, eggplants, tobacco) might have to be eliminated by those who have joint pains associated with their consumption. And there are certain foods (beef, pork and dairy, for example) that are proinflammatory: that is, they increase the inflammatory response due to their content of certain types of fats that increase the body's production of certain proinflammatory hormones called prostaglandins. Other foods, like fish, flax and hempseed, are anti-inflammatory in that they have the reverse effect. Moreover, the foods in the prohibited category are the most allergenic and therefore the most likely to aggravate the inflammatory response. If you are not sure what foods or substances you might be allergic to, see a natural health care provider. You will find the menu

Fish, flax and hemp seed oils act as anti-inflammatory agents in the body.

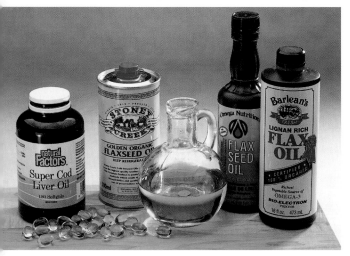

suggestions and recipes that are included in this book helpful in planning your dietary transition.

Allowed Foods and Beverages
(provided you are not allergic to them)

- Carotene-containing foods like sweet potatoes, carrots, spinach, cantaloupe, kale, squash and pumpkin
- Rice cakes, rice cereals and rice crackers
- Vitamin C- and antioxidant-containing foods like citrus fruits, broccoli, strawberries, melons, Brussels sprouts and cabbages
- Popcorn (no butter or salt added)
- Buckwheat, quinoa, corn or rice pasta
- All fresh fruits and dried fruits, preferably organic
- Lamb, poultry, fish and seafood, preferably organic (they must be well cooked)
- Organic fruit juices (freshly juiced)
- Soy, rice or almond milk
- Small amounts of nuts (except peanuts and cashews)
- Sunflower and pumpkin seeds
- Pure, filtered or ozonated water (It is important for adults to drink at least eight large glasses each day.)

What to Avoid

- Wheat and other gluten-containing grains (barley, oats, rye, spelt, amaranth, millet and kamut)
- Milk and other commercially processed milk dairy products
- Eggs
- Sugar
- Artificial sweeteners (stevia is a good non-sugar sweetener)
- All alcoholic beverages including beer and wine
- Caffeine (coffee, regular tea, colas, chocolate)
- Soft drinks and tap water (unless filtered by reverse osmosis or ozonated)
- All foods containing artificial flavorings, additives and preservatives
- Beef, pork, cold cuts, fried foods and salty foods
- Coconut
- Peanuts, cashews and their products

Essential Fatty Acids

Saturated animal fats and arachidonic acid (from red meats and dairy products) increase the inflammatory response by stimulating the production of inflammatory prostaglandins and leukotrienes.

Prostaglandins are short-lived, hormone-like substances made by the body from essential fatty acids. They are produced in response to stimulatory events such as infection, trauma, allergy or toxin exposure. They regulate blood pressure, inflammatory responses, insulin sensitivity, immune responses, tissue building (anabolic) and tissue destroying (catabolic) processes, and hundreds of other biochemical reactions.

The body makes both proinflammatory and anti-inflammatory prostaglandins depending upon the available amounts of various essential fatty acids obtained from the diet. Supplementation with flax seed oil, evening primrose oil and hemp seed oil will ensure an adequate intake of the essential fatty acids that stimulate the synthesis of the anti-inflammatory prostaglandins that block the pain and inflammatory effects of chemical mediators like leukotriene.

> Supplementing the diet with unrefined oils will ensure adequate intake of essential fatty acids.

22

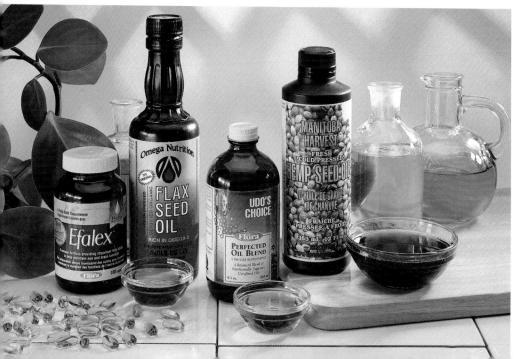

An alternate way of obtaining anti-inflammatory essential fatty acids from the diet is to eat cold-water fish such as salmon, trout, mackerel, sardines, swordfish, shark, cod and halibut. These fish contain high concentrations of omega-3 fatty acids, which have also been documented to blunt the inflammatory or allergic response. If you don't like fish, or if it's hard to find good fish, supplementation with fish oil capsules is an alternative. Good vegetarian sources of essential fatty acids are walnuts, pecans, avocados, macadamia nuts, pumpkin seeds, sesame seeds and almonds.

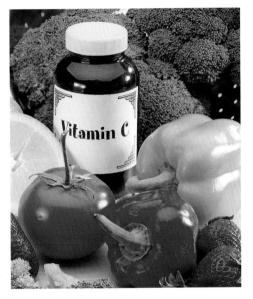

High doses of vitamin C, and eating vitamin C-rich foods, are helpful in the treatment of rheumatoid arthritis.

Antioxidants

Since the inflammatory response creates oxidative damage to tissues, the use of antioxidants helps prevent the damage that leads to permanent dysfunction. Antioxidant supplements include vitamins like natural carotenoids (carotenes, lycopenes and others), vitamin A (retinol), bioflavonoids and the proanthocyanidins (grape seed extract, pine bark extract or pycnogenols), vitamins C and E, sulfur containing amino acids like cysteine, N-acetyl-cysteine, methionine and glutathione.

Other important antioxidants with reported benefits for rheumatoid arthritis are coenzyme Q_{10} and NADH (both coenzymes found naturally in the body), as well as B-complex vitamins (especially folic acid and vitamin B_{12}), selenium and zinc. So-called superfoods like spirulina, chlorella, bee pollen, royal jelly and herbs of many different kinds have also been advocated. Whole-leaf aloe vera juice also contains high levels of many natural antioxidants.

Studies also indicate that high doses of vitamin C and bioflavonoids are helpful in the treatment of many autoimmune conditions. Bioflavonoids such as rutin, hesperidin, catechin, quercetin, pycnogenols and bilberry in high doses help strengthen the walls of capillaries thereby preventing bruising (purpura).

They stabilize the mast cell membranes and thus block the series of reactions that are associated with almost any allergy. Allergies release chemicals that damage joints, ligaments and arteries. Taking bioflavonoids will reduce vasculitis and fatigue, all symptoms of RA.

Hydrochloric Acid

Most autoimmune diseases are associated with a lack or insufficiency of hydrochloric acid production by the stomach. Achlorhydria (no acid) or hypochlohydria (low acid) leads to dozens of nutrient deficiencies. Most high-protein foods need acid for digestion. Amino acids, vitamins and minerals are poorly absorbed if acid is low or absent. The most recognized nutrient deficiency caused by low or deficient stomach acid is vitamin B_{12} deficiency, which leads to pernicious anemia and can usually only be rectified by regular vitamin B_{12} injections.

Low stomach acid may be the result of heredity, extended use of drugs (antacids, antiulcer medications), infection in the gut, or food allergies (especially to milk, dairy and wheat products). And hydrochloric acid secretion decreases with age. One study showed that by age sixty over half the population has low stomach acidity. Low hydrochloric acid can be corrected by supplementing with stomach acidifiers like glutamic acid hydrochloride, betaine and pepsin hydrochloride, apple cider vinegar, lemon juice or stomach bitters. Also helpful in this respect are pantothenic acid (vitamin B_5), vitamin C, para amino benzoic acid (PABA) and vitamin B_6.

The most accurate and reliable way to diagnose hypo-chlorhydria is with a gastric pH test using a Heidelberg capsule. This test involves having the patient swallow a capsule, which transmits pH data to a machine (radio telemetry) before and after challenges with alkaline and acid supplements. However, few physicians use the Heidelberg test owing to its cost and other logistic factors.

Another way to test for hypochlorhydria is to make use of one of the components of the comprehensive stool and digestive analysis (CSDA). The presence of a lot of undigested meat, poultry or fish fibers in a subject's stool is indirect evidence of low hydrochloric acid output by the stomach. The CSDA is done by several labs in the US. Natural health care practitioners also use livecell microscopy to demonstrate a problem with low stomach acidity. See the appendix for further information on these tests.

The enzyme bromelain, which is derived from pineapple, helps digest protein and works as an anti-inflammatory.

Enzymes

Pancreatin (animal-based pancreatic digestive enzymes), plant enzymes and bromelain (from pineapples) not only help with protein digestion in the gastrointestinal tract but have been demonstrated to work as anti-inflammatory substances as well. They also help reduce the number of proinflammatory chemical mediators like some prostaglandins and leukotrienes. The combination of bromelain, papain (from papaya), amylase, lipase, trypsin, chymotrypsin and pancreatin has been documented to be a very effective alternative to conventional anti-inflammatory drugs. This combination can be found in the digestive enzyme supplement Digeston, manufactured by Phytogenics (see "Sources").

Herbs

Curcumin is the yellow pigment of the herb turmeric. In some studies it has been reported to be as effective as cortisone without any of the associated side effects. Curcumin is primarily effective as a natural anti-inflammatory agent but it also has important uses in cancer prevention, liver disorders, heart disease and irritable bowel syndrome.

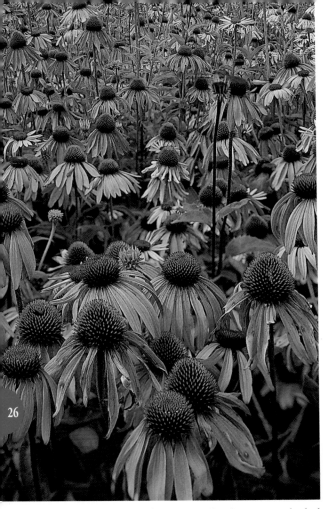

Echinacea is a highly effective herbal treatment to fight pain and inflammation.

Echinacea *(Echinacea angustifolia)* is a very popular North American herb used to treat a variety of symptoms and diseases. It has anti-inflammatory properties, and as such it has a valid and often very effective role to play in all autoimmune diseases. High doses of echinacea for extended periods of time can reduce pain just about anywhere. It is an unproven myth that echinacea is contraindicated in the treatment of rheumatoid arthritis and other autoimmune diseases. On the contrary, large doses taken for months on end are effective at modulating a hyperactive immune system.

Ginger *(Zingiber officinale)* is not only a good treatment for nausea and motion sickness but has a natural anti-inflammatory effect in arthritis, bursitis and other musculoskeletal ailments. It tones the cardiovascular system and reduces platelet aggregation similar to aspirin. One to two grams of powdered ginger a day is an average dose, but some with inflammatory conditions need higher doses taken over several months. If a burning sensation develops in the stomach, take ginger with food.

Black Cohosh *(Cimicifuga)* has traditionally been used for pain, muscular spasms and muscular and uterine inflammatory processes. Cimicifuga is useful for arthritis as well as traumatic injuries to the muscles and/or joints. Black cohosh root contains salicin, an anti-inflammatory that relieves muscle and joint pain.

Yucca *(Yucca baccata)* is used by the indigenous people of North and South America for relief of rheumatic pain. Yucca is high in saponins, which have been shown to have an anti-inflammatory action on rheumatoid arthritis.

Chaparral (*Larrea tridentata*) is common in southwestern United States as well as Mexico, and has potent anti-inflammatory and antioxidant properties that make it capable of inhibiting pro-inflammatory compounds often elevated in the synovial fluid of arthritis sufferers.

Devil's Claw (*Harpagophytum procumbens*) is a South African plant used as an arthritis remedy. Devil's claw was observed to have an action comparable to that of phenylbutazone (a NSAID) in several European studies. Besides anti-inflammatory glycosides, devil's claw also contains numerous complex constituents including the phytosterols, B-sitosterol and stigmasterol, unsaturated fatty acids, triterpenes and flavonoids.

Stinging Nettle (*Urtica dioica*) has long been recognized as an effective treatment for arthritis and gout. It can stimulate the body to excrete uric acid, a substance that can form stones and arthritic joints. Stinging nettle contains several medicinal ingredients, including acetylcholine and histamine, which are involved in pain control. Extracts of stinging nettle applied topically can help in reducing the pain caused by any kind of arthritis.

Often times a combination of natural remedies can be effective in the treatment of rheumatoid arthritis.

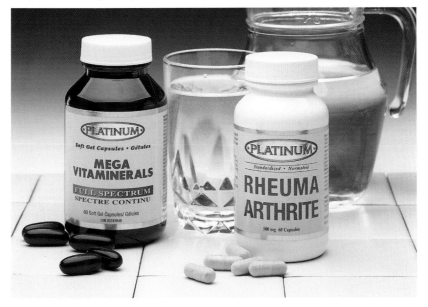

Natural Remedies for Rheumatoid Arthritis

The following is a list of various natural remedies that have been reported to be effective in the treatment of rheumatoid arthritis and other autoimmune diseases:

- Alfalfa: six or more capsules daily
- Amino acids (especially histidine): 500 mg three times daily
- Bromelain: 125–450 mg three times daily
- Plant or pancreatic proteolytic enzymes: two or more capsules with meals
- Capsicum (cayenne pepper extract): topical use only
- Cat's claw: one to three tsp tincture daily
- Coenzyme Q10: 400 mg daily
- Curcumin (turmeric extract): 500 mg three times daily
- Devil's claw: 500 mg three times daily
- Feverfew: 250 mg three times daily
- Garlic: 4,000 mcg or more daily
- Ginger: 500–1000 mg daily
- White oak: 500 mg three times daily
- White willow bark: 500 mg three times daily
- Yucca (saponin extract): four tablets or two tbsp daily
- Silica gel: two tbsp daily, or Vegesil (siicon extract from spring horsetail), or horsetail herbal tea
- Sea cucumber (bêche-de-mer): three capsules or more daily

The Leaky Gut Connection

Autoimmune diseases have been linked to a general condition known as the leaky gut syndrome. A "leaky" gut is one in which the intestinal lining is more permeable than normal. In simple terms, this means that larger than optimal spaces are present between the cells of the gut wall, thereby allowing the entrance of bacteria, fungi, parasites, toxins, undigested protein, fat and waste material into the bloodstream. These substances, which are normally not absorbed in a healthy state, pass through a damaged, hyperpermeable or leaky gut.

The leaky gut syndrome is brought about by inflammation of the gut lining. Inflammation causes the spaces between the cells to enlarge, allowing the absorption of large protein molecules. Normally these molecules would be broken down into much smaller pieces before absorption through the small spaces between the gut lining cells. The immune system starts making antibodies against the larger molecules because it recognizes these as foreign, invading substances; thus, antibodies are suddenly being made against the proteins and the previously well-tolerated foods.

These food antibodies can get into various tissues and trigger an inflammatory reaction when the corresponding food is consumed. This occurs because body tissues have antigenic sites very similar to those on food, bacteria, parasites, candida or fungi. Autoantibodies are thus created, and inflammation can become chronic. If this inflammation occurs in a joint, autoimmune arthritis develops.

Supplementing with Glutamine

Glutamine (or L-glutamine) is an amino acid supplement that helps repair leaky gut syndrome. Glutamine is the most abundant amino acid in the body and makes up more than 50 percent of the protein found in cells. For many reasons, it is an excellent healing supplement for just about anyone suffering from RA.

Stress and inflammation increases the body's demand for glutamine. Studies have shown that supplementing glutamine can prevent muscle wasting, weight loss and other common problems encountered by victims of RA. Moreover, low glutamine levels impair the immune system and increase susceptibility to infection.

Glutamine is produced primarily in skeletal muscle. Its mechanism of action is to work as an inter-organ nitrogen and carbon transporter. Glutamine is traditionally classified as a non-essential amino acid because it can be made in the body from other amino acids. Regardless of this classification, glutamine is essential for maintaining intestinal function, immune response and amino acid homeostasis during times of severe stress, as with rheumatoid arthritis. Glutamine is an important metabolic fuel for all the white blood cells, fibroblasts (cells involved in tissue repair and healing) and enterocytes (cells lining the gastrointestinal tract). Glutamine also functions as a precursor of other amino acids, glucose (blood sugar), purines and pyrimidines (DNA and RNA), and glutathione, the body's most important self-generated antioxidant.

Glutamine is an excellent healing supplement for those suffering with rheumatoid arthritis.

29

Dosage: 500-15,000 mg daily. Studies show that glutamine is well tolerated and without side effects in doses up to 40 grams per day.

The Parasite Connection

There is a parasite connection to many common health problems. Parasites compete with us for nutrients like vitamins, minerals and amino acids, and secrete waste products into our gut and bloodstream that are capable of causing various allergic and autoimmune reactions.

While rheumatoid arthritis is not necessarily caused by parasites, their presence in the body can certainly aggravate the signs and symptoms, making full recovery difficult.

There are many documented cases of rheumatoid arthritis that have actually been triggered by parasitic infection. A parasite connection needs to be considered, especially in those cases with atypical joint diseases, particularly if symptoms also include some kind of gastrointestinal upset (diarrhea, constipation, bloating and gas) that will not go away.

If you have rheumatoid arthritis and are not doing well with either conventional or natural treatments, visit a natural health care provider and get tested for parasites. This is best done through testing by a lab specializing in parasite detection (e.g., Great Smokies Medical Laboratory, Meridian Valley Clinical Laboratory; see the appendix). The treatment of parasites with diet, herbs, enzymes and even prescription drugs may be an important factor to consider as part of the treatment of resistant cases of rheumatoid arthritis.

Antifungal Regimes and Probiotics

Autoimmune diseases often respond to antifungal treatments. Evidence exists that fungi, through their production of mycotoxins, initiate many autoimmune diseases by triggering inflammation in the gastrointestinal tract, which in turn leads to the development of the leaky gut syndrome. Diseases of "unknown etiology" often have a fungal connection, with treatment of the fungal infection bringing about an improvement or elimination of that disease.

In treating any fungal infection, it is important to realize that many foods, even those considered to be healthy, are heavily colonized by fungi and their mycotoxins. These include corn, peanuts, cashews and dried coconuts. To a lesser degree, fungi can also be found in barley, rye, wheat, rice, millet and practically all cereal grains. A diet high in contaminated grains and nuts increases the likelihood of fungal colonization of the gastrointestinal tract. Worse, animals fed mycotoxin-contaminated grains end up with fungal overgrowth. This is evidenced by the fact that the fat and muscles of most grain-fed animals in North America are loaded with mycotoxins. While it cannot be said that fungi and their mycotoxins cause fibromyalgia, there are numerous reports that the use of antifungal remedies clears or improves many cases of this condition.

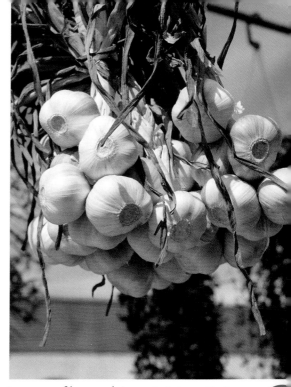

Garlic is an effective antifungal remedy.

Diet is very important in the treatment of any fungal infection. Sugar feeds fungi and must be eliminated from the diet. This includes maple syrup, honey, molasses and fruit juice. In severe infections, even whole fruits should be eliminated for several weeks. Milk, white-flour products, foods containing yeast, peanuts, mushrooms, melons and moldy foods (e.g., leftovers) all contribute to worsening any fungal infection. Some well documented natural antifungal remedies include probiotics like *Lactobacillus acidophilus* and *bifidus*, garlic, extract of wild oregano oil, caprylic acid, olive leaf extract, colloidal silver and tea tree oil. Some individuals respond poorly to the natural approach and are only helped by prescription antifungal drugs (e.g., nystatin, itraconazole, fluconazole and others).

Supplementation with probiotic products provides another unique type of protection against some of the microbes reported to trigger RA. Probiotics is the name given to the "friendly" bacteria that maintain a healthy intestinal flora, an essential aspect of overall health.

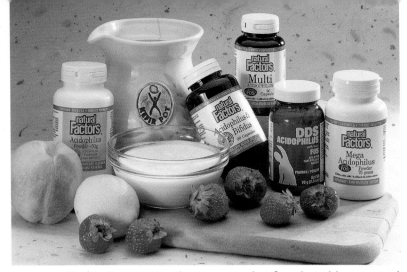

Probiotics provide protection against some of the microbes reported to trigger rheumatoid arthritis.

Probiotics prevent the overgrowth of undesirable intestinal bacteria and micro-organisms that produce toxins. If harmful bacteria dominate the intestines, essential vitamins and enzymes are not produced, and the level of harmful substances rises, leading to the development of the leaky gut syndrome and subsequent RA.

Well-known probiotics include *Lactobacillus acidophilus* and *Bifidobacterium bifidum*. Another probiotic that has recently generated a great deal of interest is the friendly yeast known as *Saccharomyces boulardii*, an organism that belongs to the brewer's yeast family. *S. boulardii* is not a permanent resident of the intestine, but taken orally it produces lactic acid and some B vitamins, and has an overall immune-enhancing effect.

Probiotics are considered to be very safe and well tolerated in the usual dosages prescribed.

Highly sensitive individuals have reported the occasional occurrence of indigestion (nausea, heartburn) that disappeared when the supplement was discontinued or the brand of probiotic was changed.

Sugar, caffeine, alcohol, chlorine, tobacco, prescription antibiotics, steroids, vaccinations and x-rays inhibit probiotics. There is also some evidence that casein, a milk protein found in most commercial dairy products, inhibits probiotic growth. The antibiotics found in dairy products are also a factor in suppressing probiotics. A diet high in complex carbohydrates (vegetables, fruits, whole grains, legumes) encourages the proliferation of most probiotics.

Nondigestible food factors that selectively stimulate the growth and activity of probiotics in the gut are referred to as "prebiotics." The best example of a prebiotic is FOS (fructo-oligo-saccharides). This substance is found naturally in many vegetables, grains and fruits, including Jerusalem artichokes, chicory, burdock, garlic and onions. In Japan, FOS is widely used as a sweetener.

Cultured dairy products like yogurt, acidophilus milk, buttermilk, sour cream, cottage cheese and kefir are the best-known sources of friendly bacteria. Equally effective probiotic sources include cultured/fermented soy products like soymilk, tofu, tempeh and miso. Other, lesser-known food sources of probiotics are sauerkraut and sourdough breads. If dietary sources are not easily available, supplemental probiotic powders and capsules are good alternatives.

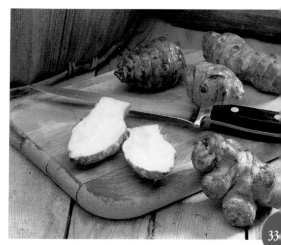

33

FOS, which stimulates the growth of probiotics in the gut, is derived from Jerusalem artichokes.

Hormonal Therapies

Rheumatoid arthritis and other autoimmune diseases have been reported to respond in varying degrees to DHEA (dehydroepiandrosterone), pregnenolone, cortisol, estrogen, progesterone, testosterone and thyroid hormones. DHEA is an effective natural treatment for most types of arthritis due to its ability to modulate the inflammatory response.

DHEA is the most abundant androgen (male hormone) produced by the adrenal cortex of both males and females. It can be found in almost any organ including the testes, the ovaries, the lungs and the brain. Testosterone is synthesized from DHEA in both males and females. One of the theories as to why women are more likely to get rheumatoid arthritis and other autoimmune diseases is because of their relatively lower levels of DHEA and testosterone. Natural precursors to DHEA can be found in wild yam but studies do not indicate that this is equivalent to the pure hormone. Testosterone can be used if DHEA fails to produce positive results.

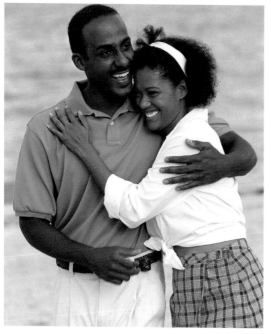

Women may be more susceptible than men to rheumatoid arthritis because of their lower levels of DHEA, the male hormone.

The Safety Controversy

While it is true that the long-term effects of daily DHEA supplementation are not fully known, the same can be said for many of the prescription and non-prescription drugs given quick approval without long-term safety and efficacy studies. According to reports from the Office of Technology Assessment, about 80 percent of all currently available medications on the market have never been subjected to clinical trials. Americans who eat the typical commercially available dairy products, chicken, pork and beef products consume plenty of steroid hormones, antibiotics and a long list of other drugs.

The public, with full US Food and Drug Administration (FDA) approval (Health Protection Branch or HPB in Canada), can self-medicate with unproven over-the-counter antibiotic creams, anti-yeast drugs, eye drops, cortisone creams and inhalers, stimulants, antihistamines, antifungal treatments, sleeping aids and many other potentially harmful chemicals. A long list of readily available synthetic steroids, birth control pills and fertility drugs have been linked to higher rates of cancer. The long-term use of non-steroidal anti-inflammatory drugs (NSAIDS) has been associated with as many as 25,000 cases of gastrointestinal hemorrhage each year. So, let's put the toxicity issue into perspective.

Some of the short-term side effects of FDA-approved, freely available drugs include yeast infections and resistant bacterial strains (antibiotic overuse), gastrointestinal hemorrhage (NSAIDS), breast cancer, thromboembolism and stroke (birth control pills), and heart attacks (antihistamines combined with antibiotics or antifungal drugs). None of the short-term side effects of DHEA come even remotely close to this. In one study, a daily dose of 1,600 mg of DHEA given for twenty-eight days to healthy subjects resulted in some insulin resistance but no other noticeable side effects. DHEA studies in lupus cases where 200 mg daily was taken for over three months concluded that it was well tolerated except for mild to moderate acne and occasional mild hirsuitism (abnormal hair growth). There is no evidence that DHEA is any more harmful than the birth control pill (a steroid) or over-the-counter cortisone (steroid) creams, lotions, eye or ear drops.

Although the long-term effects of DHEA are not fully known, those of many over-the-counter and prescription drugs in the US are well known but still left alone by the FDA. For example, many cough, cold and flu remedies containing ephedrine or pseude-phedrine can worsen or even create high blood pressure, urinary flow restriction and prostate problems in men as well as heart beat irregularities, panic attacks, strokes and sudden deaths from heart attacks. Long-term side effects of some FDA approved diet pills can cause pulmonary hypertension and respiratory failure. The long-term use of calcium channel blockers have recently been reported to cause sudden death and yet these drugs were put on the market without any consideration for long-term effects. Despite the growing horror stories about the toxicity of calcium channel blockers, antidepressants and immunosuppressant drugs, the FDA makes no attempt to take them off the market. The belief that just because they are under a doctor's prescription they are safe is an unjustified one. The FDA has also done nothing to curtail the availability of nicotine and alcohol products that kill millions of Americans each year.

The truth is that compared to the majority of over-the-counter drugs, hormones and food supplements, DHEA administration is relatively safe. However, until more is known about its long-term effects, DHEA should be used with caution.

Hormone Levels

Please also note that before supplementing with any hormonal remedies, it's important to obtain lab testing to verify low hormone levels. Research shows that saliva testing is more accurate than blood tests for assessing hormone levels. This is because steroid hormones like DHEA are carried around the bloodstream complexed with a carrier protein. The active hormone is "free," meaning that it does not have a protein carrier. Blood tests do not distinguish between the free and the bound form of the hormone, while the saliva test only measures the free (active) hormone. It is therefore a more accurate reflection of that hormone's activity.

Some labs in the US offer saliva testing directly to the public, thereby avoiding the need to consult a doctor. (See "Sources" for further information.) If you feel more comfortable working with your doctor, he or she can order and interpret saliva testing for you.

Unlike American consumers, Canadians need a prescription to obtain DHEA, natural progesterone and other natural hormones. The tests, however, are available to anyone without a doctor's approval and are a good first step in optimizing your hormone levels.

Other Immune System Regulators . . . .
Vitamin E

In low doses (under 800 IU per day), vitamin E may have little or no effect on autoimmune disease; however, in doses well above 2,000 IU, vitamin E weakens (down regulates) autoimmune disease.

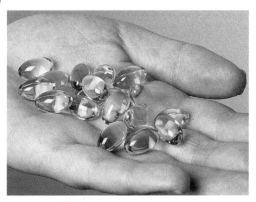

High doses of vitamin E will weaken the effects of rheumatoid arthritis.

PABA

Para amino benzoic acid (PABA) may be effective in autoimmune diseases to offset immune system hyperactivity. Dosage: 2,000-3,000 mg daily for up to six months

Colostrum

The colostrum from bovine sources is another powerful immune system modulator, able to stimulate a sluggish immune system or dampen an overactive immune response such as occurs with autoimmune diseases. Colostrum has been documented to be helpful in the treatment of autoimmune diseases like rheumatoid arthritis. It is a nutrient-rich milk precursor that contains immunoglobulins, growth factors, antimicrobial proteins and carbohydrates that transfer immunity from the mother cow to the calf's gastrointestinal system immediately following birth. Colostrum is free of milk, lactose and other allergy-inducing products.

Removal of Mercury Amalgam

In many cases of autoimmune disease, replacement of mercury with non-metal fillings is effective at reversing symptoms. Mercury may well be behind the immune system abnormalities leading to conditions like rheumatoid arthritis.

Antibiotics

The use of the antibiotic minocycline at a dose of 100 mg twice daily for several months has been shown to be effective in reversing up to 80 percent of cases of rheumatoid arthritis and other autoimmune diseases. If using minocycline or any other antibiotic, make sure that anti-fungal therapy plus a good friendly bacterial culture is also used (e.g., *Lactobacillus acidophilus* and *bifido bacteria*).

The treatment approach taken to any autoimmune disease depends on many different factors and is best individualized for the patient by a natural health care practitioner.

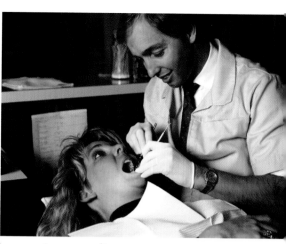

The mercury in dental fillings may be linked to the immune system abnormalities that lead to rheumatoid arthritis.

Psycho-Spiritual
Aspects of Rheumatoid Arthritis . . . .

Never underestimate the importance of the human mind and soul in creating ill health. Your state of mind can have a powerful effect, in a positive or negative way, on your health. Indeed, many people who suffer from RA report some stressful life event immediately preceding attacks of arthritis. Most frequently the stressful event involves the disruption of a meaningful relationship. Practitioners who see a lot of RA patients often talk about the "rheumatoid personality," which is described as devoid of affect, emotionally flat or colorless, fearful and socially withdrawn. While each RA personality is different, victims have often been described as compulsive, perfectionist, over-conscientious and helpful, excessively moral with suppressed or repressed resentment or hostility or having depressive tendencies. Rigidity, stubbornness, inflexibility and immobility are terms that also frequently describe those with RA.

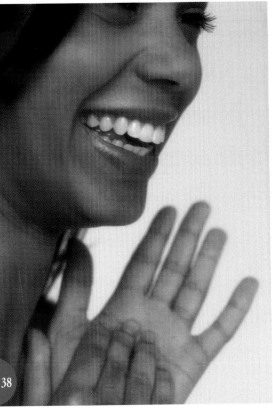

Psychological or spiritual therapies may help reduce or eliminate the inflammation associated with rheumatoid arthritis.

Non-Physical Treatments · ·

About twenty years ago, Joe W., a thirty-year-old friend of the family, was diagnosed with a severe form of RA. He went to the best specialists conventional medicine had to offer, including rheumatologists. When nothing from conventional medicine was able to have any impact on his arthritis, he consulted nutritionists, herbalists, homeopaths and even a doctor of environmental medicine (clinical ecologist in those days). For nearly two years he went through extensive testing and spent over $10,000 on various detoxification programs, chelation therapy, colonic irrigation, herbal supplements, vitamins, enzymes, allergy treatments and other remedies. Nothing worked. Finally, a close friend asked him if he had considered the possibility of stress as a possible cause of his arthritis. This led Joe to a psychotherapist who was able to help Joe overcome the emotional stressors at the source of his arthritis. Three weeks later, the arthritis was in complete remission. There have been no flare-ups since that time.

Emotional or spiritual stress may not always be so readily curable by psychotherapy but it is definitely an area of potential help to anyone suffering from RA. If stress is indeed a trigger for RA flare-ups, psychological or spiritual therapies may be very effective in reducing or eliminating the inflammatory process. Without going into any great detail about how and why these psycho-spiritual techniques work to relieve arthritis, my observation is that they can make a huge difference for any person suffering from rheumatoid arthritis.

Some of the modalities I have seen work well for RA victims over the past two decades are prayer, religious worship, psychodynamic psychotherapy, biofeedback, behavior modification, group therapy, hypnosis, guided imagery, visualization and affirmations.

Psychologists, psycho-neuro-immunologists and other holistic healers too numerous to list have proven the immense value of visualization, positive thinking and prayer in treating practically all diseases, especially cancer, heart disease and autoimmune diseases like RA. One visualizes tumor cells being gobbled up by the white cells and guess what? The cancer is better controlled. Knowing what coenzyme Q_{10} and hawthorn does for high blood pressure and visualizing how these remedies work will produce more positive results in blood pressure control than the biochemical effects of these substances on their own.

So it is with RA. Visualize the essential fatty acid supplements and the massive vitamin E doses turning off the abnormal inflammatory response and the arthritic process weakens. In other words, the more you know about the therapy and how it works, the better are the treatment results in the long run. Using this type of visualization can work wonders. Just the very fact that you are reading this book has already set off an unconscious healing process. If you feel better just reading this book, it is because you have taken a positive step toward better health by seeking help beyond that offered by conventional medical approaches. You are beginning to take control.

In her book, *You Can Heal Your Life*, Louise Hay suggests several affirmations for RA to be repeated several times each day for at least forty days in a row. Reciting affirmations, going to church or receiving psychotherapy may not be for everyone. If it does not feel right to you, it probably isn't. Forcing yourself to follow a therapy that you are not comfortable with can be more detrimental than the disease process itself. Choose another way to get in touch with your emotions and spiritual life. There are many choices. Whatever you try should align with your beliefs, not someone else's, and it should be positive and uplifting.

The psychological approaches outlined above combined with the protocols discussed throughout this book will give you the tools you need to restore your health. It will take time and commitment and the results will vary between individuals: not everyone with RA will achieve complete remission. At the very least, however, you will gain better control of your condition: by no longer seeing yourself as its victim you take the upper hand and steer a course toward better health.

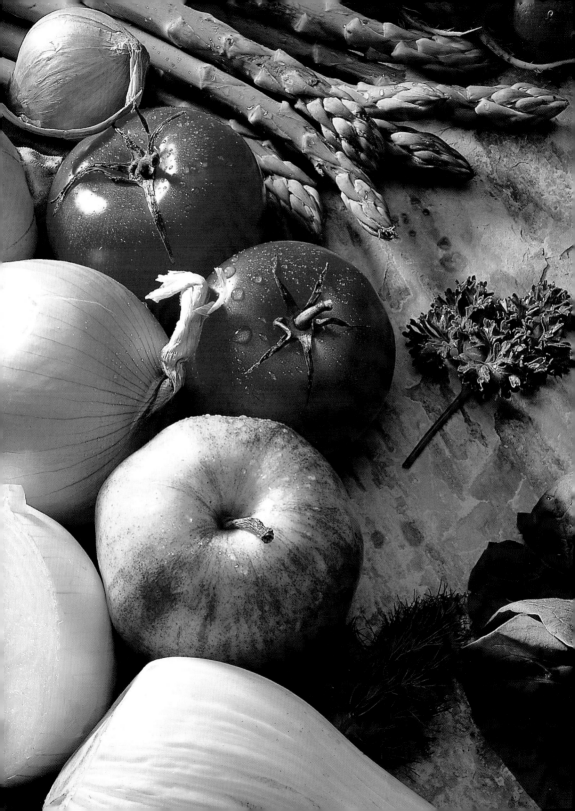

Following an allergy-free diet will bring the most dramatic benefits to those suffering from rheumatoid arthritis.

Raw Sauerkraut Salad with Flax Oil

Raw sauerkraut is one of the best vegetable sources of lactic acid, which is very beneficial for intestinal health. It can be bought in health food stores and delicatessens but the best sauerkraut is the kind you make at home. See *The Cultured Cabbage* by Klaus Kaufmann (*alive* books, 1998) for simple instructions for homemade sauerkraut. Only unrefined flax seed oil will make this dish a delicacy.

2 cups raw sauerkraut
(such as Eden brand)

2 tbsp onion, finely chopped

2 medium-size dill pickles, finely chopped

4 tbsp flax oil

Chopped parsley for garnish

Chop the sauerkraut into short strands then add onion and dill pickle and mix with flax oil. Garnish with parsley and serve.

Serves 4

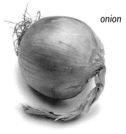

onion

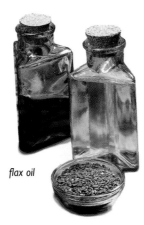

flax oil

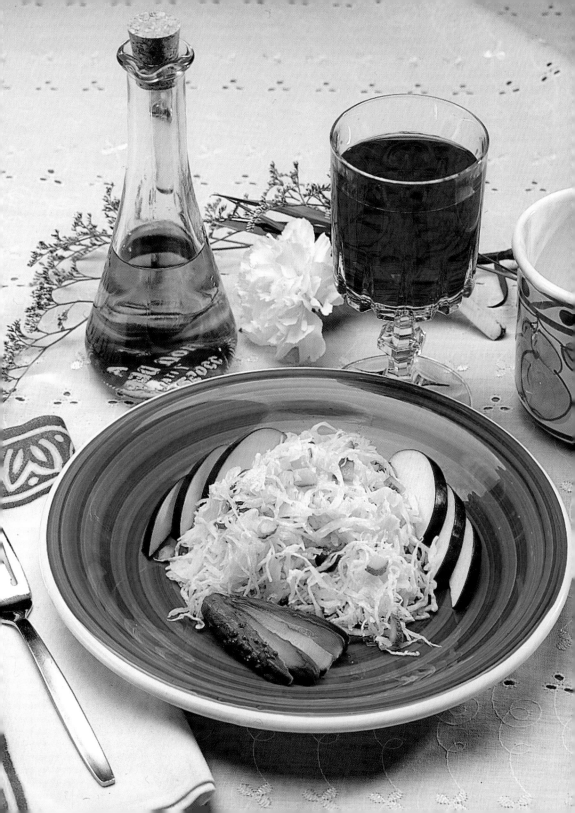

Mulligatawny Soup

There's an extra dose of the natural anti-inflammatory agent, curcumin, in this flavorful and warming soup. The curcumin in the turmeric is usually what gives curry power its rich yellow color. By the way, the spice cumin also contains some curcumin.

1 cup (250 ml) **chickpeas, cooked**

½ cup (125 ml) **onion, minced**

½ cup (125 ml) **carrot, diced**

½ cup (125 ml) **celery, diced**

1½ cups (375 ml) **turnip, diced**

2 tbsp extra-virgin olive oil

2 tsp curry powder

Pinch cayenne pepper

Pinch ground cumin

Pinch ground coriander

Sea salt, to taste

2 ½ cups (625 ml) **vegetable stock**

1 tbsp butter

⅔ cup (165 ml) **apple, peeled and grated**

Fresh parsley, chopped, for garnish

Purée the chickpeas.

In a large pot, heat oil over medium heat and sauté onion, carrot, celery and turnip for 5 minutes. Add spices, salt and sauté for 2 minutes. Add vegetable stock, butter, apple and cooked chickpeas; cover and simmer until vegetables are tender. Garnish with parsley and serve.

Serves 2

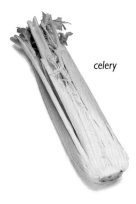

celery

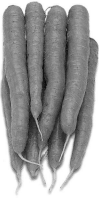

carrot

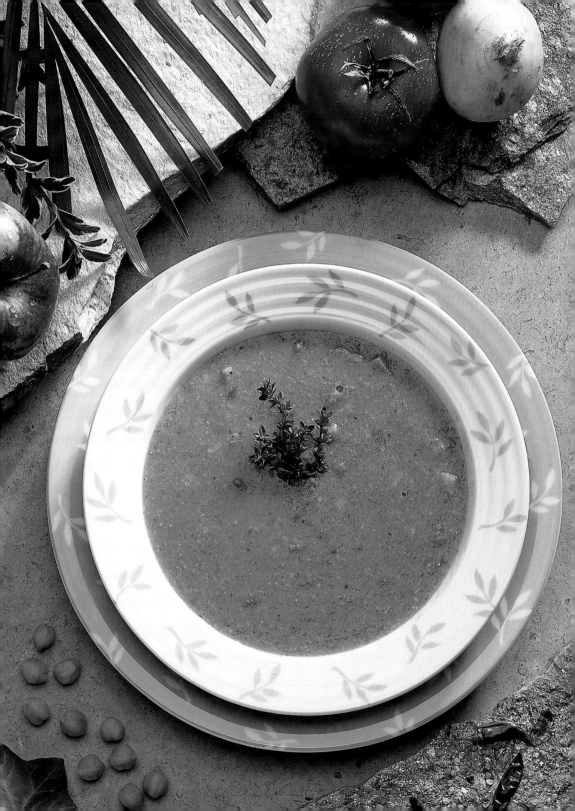

Jicama-Yam Soup with Chips

The sweet yam and jicama make a rich and nutritious soup that's easily digested. Yam is an excellent source of carotene among other antioxidants that work to prevent arthritic inflammation.

1 yam, peeled

1 small white onion, diced

2 cloves garlic, minced

1 medium jicama, peeled and cubed

2 tbsp + 2 tbsp extra-virgin olive oil

2 cups (500 ml) **water**

1 cup (250 ml) **rice milk**

2 tbsp ginger, minced

1 tbsp lemon grass, chopped

2 tsp cilantro, chopped

Dice half the yam and cut the other half in wedges.

To prepare the soup, heat 2 tablespoons of oil in a pot over medium heat and sauté onion, garlic, jicama and diced yam until soft. Add water, rice milk, ginger and lemon grass; cover and simmer for 5 to 7 minutes. Remove from heat, pour soup into a blender and purée until smooth. You can pour the soup through a sieve for an even smoother consistency. Return soup to the pot, stir in cilantro and keep warm.

In the meantime, heat 2 tablespoons of oil in a pan over medium heat and sauté the yam wedges until golden brown. Serve with the soup.

Serves 2

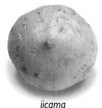

jicama

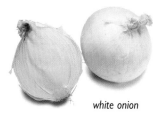

white onion

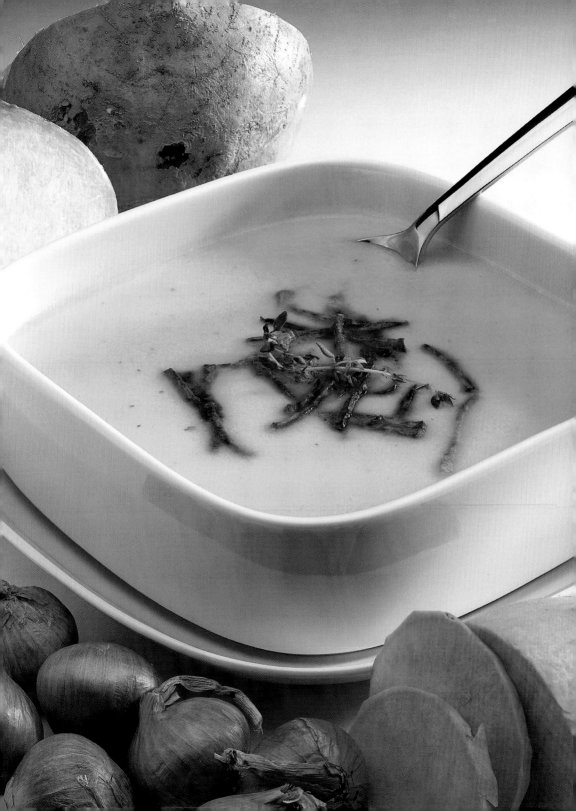

Fruity Arugula Salad

Emphasize raw fruits and vegetables for a diet low in protein and calories, and rich in the nutrients needed for rebuilding. The arugula and fruit provide the antioxidant vitamins C and E that reduce inflammation and maintain and build cartilage. The essential fats in the walnut oil also help reduce inflammation as well as lubricate joints, generate bone material and stimulate digestion.

1 lb (500 g) **arugula**

1 cup (250 ml) **black plums, cut in wedges**

1 cup (250 ml) **peaches, cut in wedges**

½ cup (125 ml) **blackberries**

Dressing:

4 tbsp walnut or hazelnut oil

Juice of ½ cup (125 ml) **blackberries**

1 tsp wheat-free tamari

Sea salt and fresh ground pepper, to taste

In a bowl, whisk together all dressing ingredients. Place arugula and fruit onto plates, drizzle dressing over top, and serve.

Serves 2

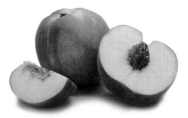

peach

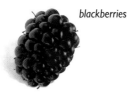

blackberries

Press the blackberries through a sieve to extract the juice then save the blackberry pulp to make jam or eat it with your breakfast cereal.

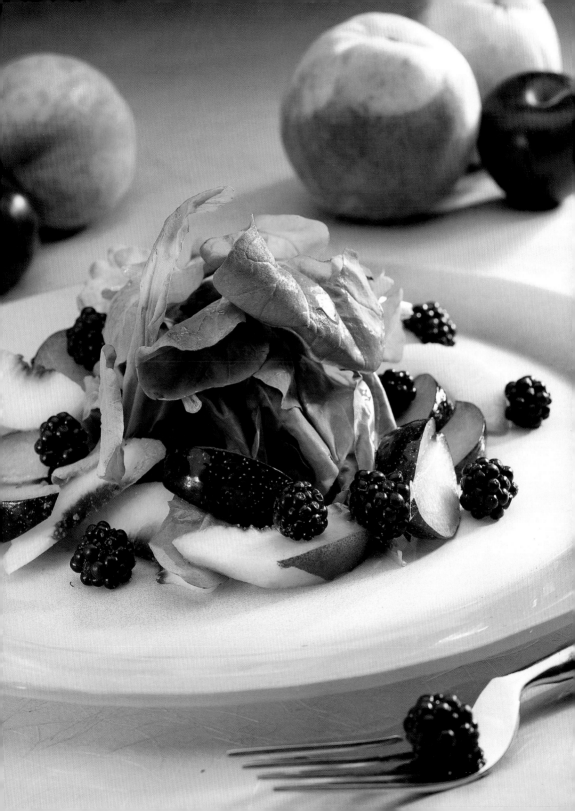

Mixed Greens
with Nectarine and Red Beet

The colors in this salad tell you that it contains a natural treasure-trove of the antioxidant vitamins helpful in treating autoimmune diseases. Greens contain high amounts of folic acid; carrots and nectarines are rich in vitamin A; red beets in vitamins A, B-complex and C; and avocado in vitamin E. You'll also get plenty of plant enzymes to help alleviate inflammation.

2 medium-sized red beets, sliced in wedges

½ lb (250 g) **organic mixed greens**

1 ripe nectarine, cut in wedges

1 ripe avocado, cut in wedges

8 slices carrot

Dressing:

3 tbsp red beet juice (reserved from cooking the beets)

2 tbsp cold-pressed flax seed oil

2 tbsp extra-virgin olive oil

1 tbsp Dijon mustard

Sea salt to taste

Bring a pot of water to a boil and cook the beets for 25 minutes on low heat. Reserving the beet juice, drain the beets and rinse them under cold water.

In a large bowl, whisk together all dressing ingredients. Set aside 1 tablespoon of dressing then toss the mixed greens with remaining dressing.

Place the greens on the center of serving plates and arrange red beet, nectarine, avocado and carrot around. Drizzle the reserved tablespoon of dressing over fruit and vegetables and serve immediately.

Serves 2

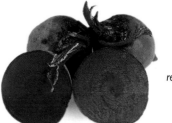

red beet

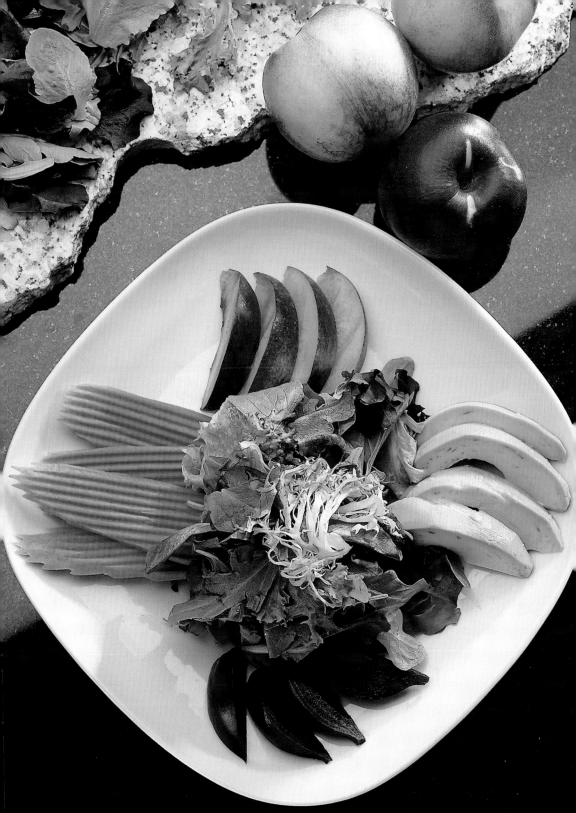

Cucumber-Avocado Soup

Simple, fast and tasty! This is especially wonderful when served cold on a hot summer day.

1 ripe avocado, cut in small chunks

2 cloves garlic, minced

1 shallot, minced

½ English cucumber, grated

1 cup (450 ml) **kefir or goat's milk yogurt**

¼ cup (250 ml) **sparkling water**

1 tbsp lime juice

2 tbsp cold-pressed hazelnut, walnut or flax oil

Fresh herbs of your choice (parsley, dill, tarragon, thyme)

Pinch ground nutmeg

Sea salt and freshly ground pepper, to taste

In a large bowl, thoroughly combine all ingredients, making sure the cucumber is not too watery. Cover and refrigerate at least 1 hour before serving.

Serves 2

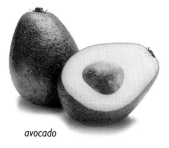

avocado

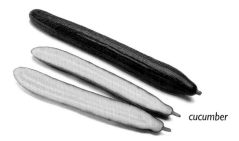

cucumber

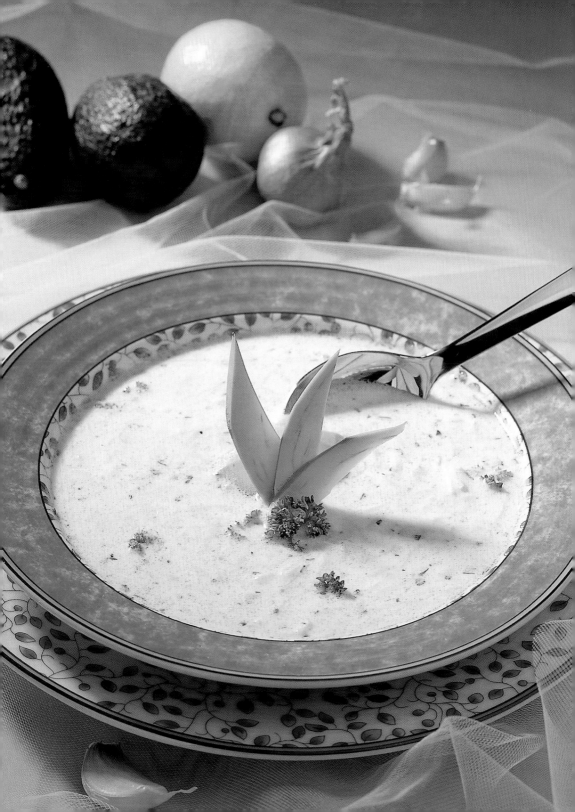

Stuffed Squash with Endive

Baked squash is comfort food and this combination of vegetables provides a bounty of beta-carotene-rich foods.

2 medium squash

2 tbsp extra-virgin olive oil

1 cup (250 ml) **turnip, cubed**

1 cup (250 ml) **Jerusalem artichoke, cubed**

1 cup (250 ml) **carrots, cubed**

2 tbsp coconut oil or extra-virgin olive oil

½ cup (125 ml) **onion, cubed**

1 cup (250 ml) **black beans, cooked**

¼ cup (60 ml) **green onions**

1 tsp fresh rosemary, chopped

1 tsp ginger

1 Belgian endive, leaves separated

Fresh cilantro, for garnish

Preheat oven to 375°F (190°C).

Cut squash in half (horizontally), remove the seeds and scoop out the flesh. Set empty squash halves aside. Cut the flesh into cubes and set aside.

Brush bottom of the squash halves with 2 tablespoons of olive oil, season with salt and pepper, then place them in an ovenproof pan and bake for 15 minutes or until tender. Keep warm.

Bring a pot of salted water to a boil and blanch cubed squash, turnip, Jerusalem artichoke and carrots for 5 minutes. Drain and immediately rinse with cold water. Set aside.

In a large pan, heat coconut oil over medium heat and sauté onion and ginger for 2 to 3 minutes. Add blanched vegetables, beans, green onion, rosemary and ginger and sauté for 2 minutes longer.

To serve, place squash cups onto plates and fill them with sautéed vegetables. Arrange endive leaves, sprinkle with cilantro and serve.

Serves 2

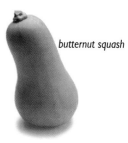

butternut squash

54

To cook black beans, soak them overnight, or for at least 2 hours, in lukewarm water. Drain and place in a pot of fresh salted water and cook for 30 to 35 minutes or until tender. Drain.

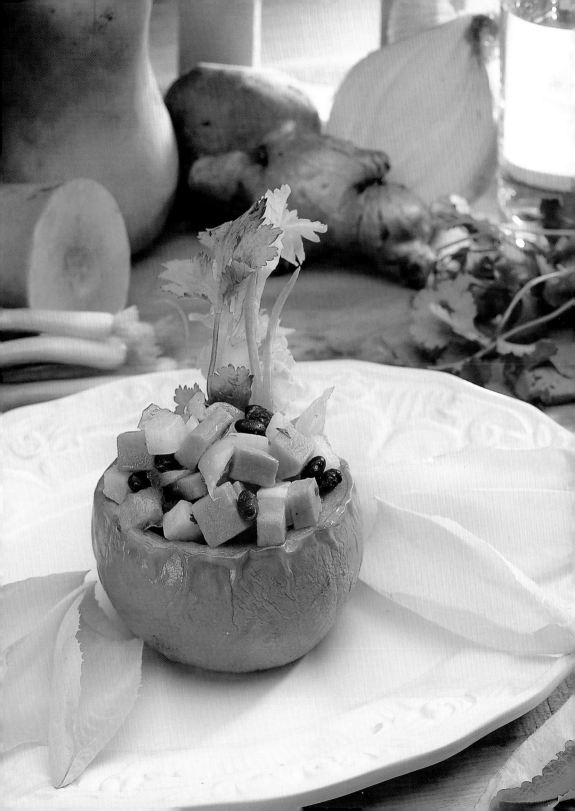

Vegetable-Rice Stew

Bursting with minerals and B vitamins, this wholesome stew will fill you up for the day.

1 cup (250 ml) **brown rice**

1½ qt (1½ L) **vegetable stock or water**

1 cup (250 ml) **onion, diced ½"** (1 cm)

3 cloves garlic, minced

2 tbsp extra-virgin olive oil

1 cup (250 ml) **carrots, diced ½"** (1 cm)

1 cup (250 ml) **turnip, diced ½"** (1 cm)

½ cup (125 ml) **fennel, cut ½"** (1 cm)

1 cup (250 ml) **celery, diced ½"** (1 cm)

1 cup (250 ml) **green beans, cut ½"** (1 cm)

1 cup (250 ml) **corn kernels**

1 cup (250 ml) **green peas**

2 bay leaves

1 tbsp Bragg's amino

Herbamare, to taste

Fresh herbs of your choice, such as rosemary, thyme or parsley, chopped

1 tbsp flax seed oil, for garnish

In a pot, cook rice in 2 cups (½ quart or 500 ml) of vegetable stock until all liquid is absorbed.

In a separate pot, heat oil and sauté onion and garlic until tender. Slowly add vegetables in this order: carrots, turnip, fennel, celery, beans, corn and peas. Sauté until tender. Add remaining vegetable stock and bay leaves. Cover and simmer for 5 minutes then add cooked rice and simmer for 5 minutes longer. Add Bragg's and season with Herbamare and fresh herbs.

Pour soup into bowls, drizzle with flax seed oil and serve.

Serves 4

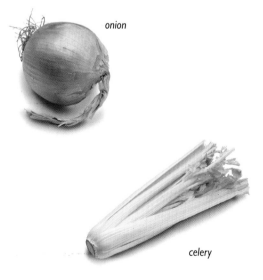

onion

celery

For more recipes using flax seed oil, read *Fantastic Flax* by Siegfried Gursche (*alive* Natural Health Guide #1).

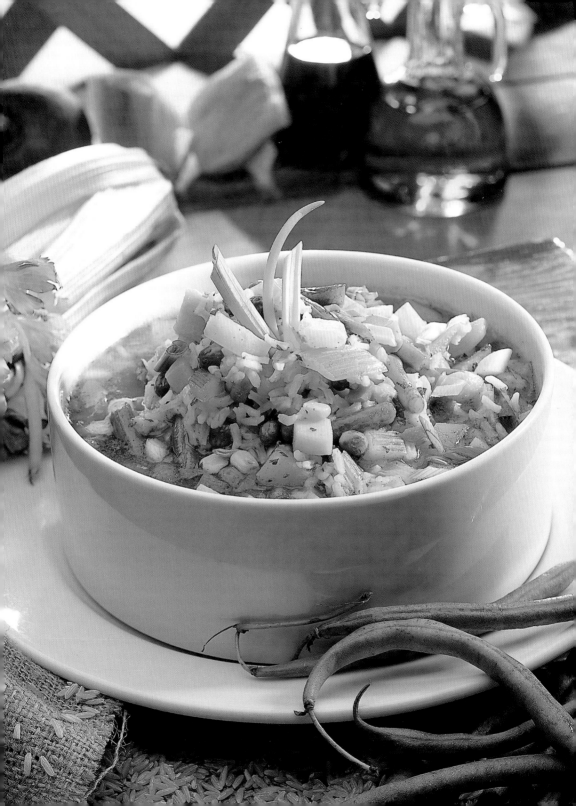

Steamed Vegetables
with Mashed Cilantro Yam

Yam is actually a type of sweet potato but is not related to potatoes of the nightshade family that often aggravate arthritis. Yam is an excellent source of antioxidants, carotenoids and vitamins A and C.

Mashed Cilantro Yam:

2 cups (450 g) **yam, cut in 1" (2.5 cm) cubes**

1 ½ cups (375 ml) **vegetable stock or water**

1 tbsp fresh cilantro, chopped

2 tsp ginger, finely minced

1 tsp garlic, finely minced

Pinch sea salt

Pinch ground allspice

Steamed Vegetables:

1 cup (250 g) **carrots, sliced**

1 cup (250 g) **broccoli florets**

1 cup (250 g) **cauliflower florets**

1 cup (250 g) **mushrooms, quartered**

Sea salt to taste

1 tbsp cold-pressed flax seed oil

1 tbsp green onions, chopped, for garnish

In a medium pot, bring the vegetable stock to a boil, add yam and cook for 15 to 18 minutes or until tender. Drain the liquid and return yam to pot. (Save the stock for another dish.) Add remaining ingredients and mash until smooth and velvety.

In the meantime, place carrots, broccoli, cauliflower and mushrooms in a bamboo steamer. Season with salt then cover and steam for 7 to 10 minutes.

Place mashed yam onto plates, arrange vegetables around and drizzle flax seed oil over top. Garnish with green onions and serve.

Serves 2

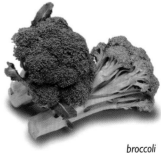

broccoli

If you don't have a bamboo steamer, use a regular steamer or blanch the vegetables in a pot of boiling water.

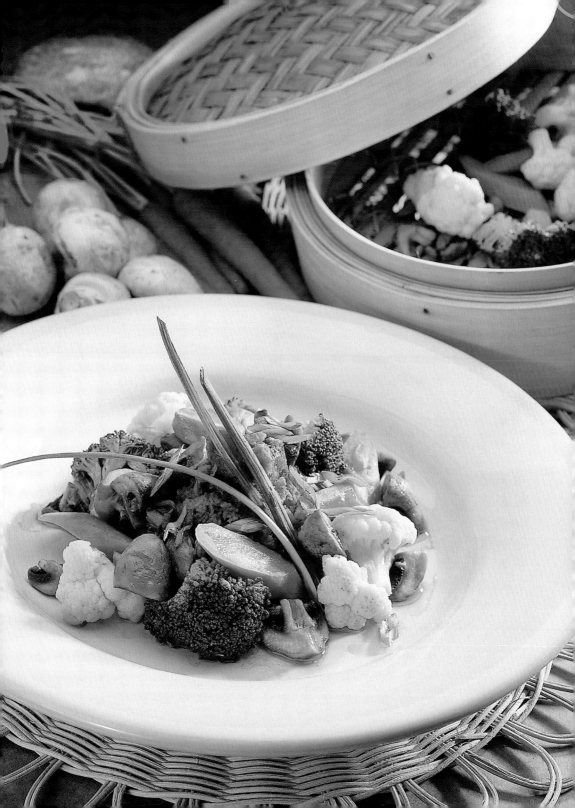

Quinoa Patties with Zucchini

Quinoa has a nutty, tasty flavor and is a good source of trace minerals. Served with the nutritious and delicious zucchini, and a red beet salad on the side, this complete meal with satisfy both your health requirements and your taste buds.

1 medium zucchini, sliced ¼" thick

1 tbsp Italian parsley or cilantro

4 tbsp green onion, chopped

4 tbsp finely chopped carrot

1 tbsp flax seed oil

¼ cup (100 ml) **olive oil**

1½ cups (350 g) **quinoa**

1 qt (1 L) **water**

1 tbsp natural, organic butter

Red Beet Salad:

3 medium red beets, cooked and cut in cubes (save the juice left from cooking)

1½ qt (1½ L) **water**

¼ cup apple cider vinegar

¼ cup maple syrup

3 cloves

1 cinnamon stick

Cook quinoa in salted water until it is soft and tender and all liquid has evaporated. In the meantime, sauté garlic, onion, and green onion in two tablespoons of the olive oil. Season this mixture with salt and pepper and add it to the cooked quinoa. Mix thoroughly and let cool. Form 3-ounce patties and sauté in the rest of olive oil until both sides are golden brown.

Brush both sides of the zucchini slices with olive oil, place them on a cookie sheet and roast it them in the oven at 380º F (190º C) for approximately 10 minutes. Arrange zucchini slices and quinoa patties on serving plates and drizzle two tablespoons of beet juice over top. Serve with red beet salad, garnished with parsley.

Cook red beet in a large pot, combine water, apple cider vinegar, maple syrup, cloves and cinnamon stick, and bring to a boil. Add the beets, cover and simmer for 45 minutes or until tender. Drain and let cool. You can cook the beets a day ahead, if you like. Before serving pour 1 tablespoon of flax seed oil over the red beet.

Serves 2

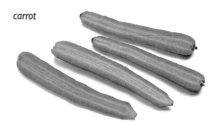

carrot

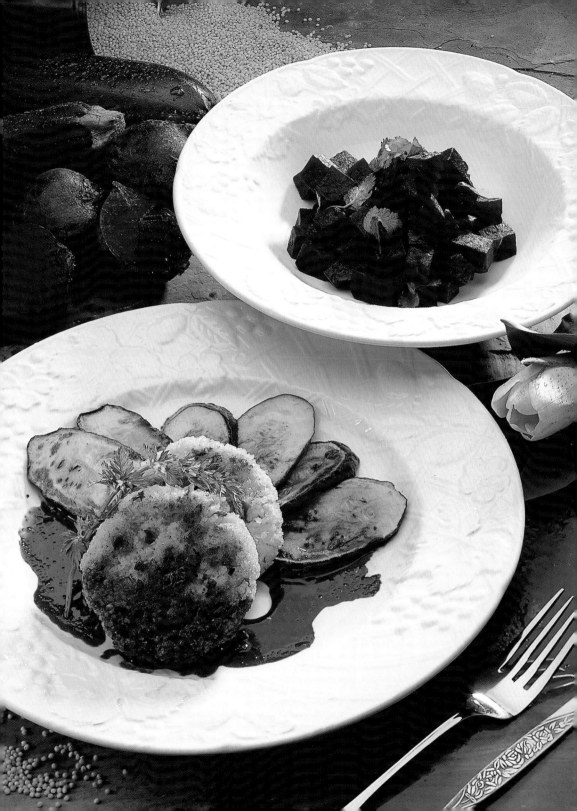

references

Barton-Wright, E. C., and W. A. Elliott. "The pantothenic acid metabolism of rheumatoid arthritis." *Lancet.* 2 (1963): 862-63.

Bjarnason, I. et al. "Intestinal permeability and inflammation in rheumatoid arthritis: Effects of non-steroidal anti-inflammatory drugs." *Lancet.* 2 (1984): 1171-4.

Gaby, Alan R. "Dehydroepiandrosterone: Biological effects and clinical significance." *Alternative Medicine Review.* Vol. 1, no. 2 (1996): 60-69.

Gottschall, Elaine. *Breaking The Vicious Cycle: Intestinal Health Through Diet.* Kirkton, ON: The Kirkton Press, 1994.

Grennan, D. M. et al. "Serum copper and zinc in rheumatoid arthritis and osteoarthritis." *New Zealand. Medical Journal.* Vol. 91, no. 652 (1980): 47-50.

Honkanen, V. et al. "Vitamins A and E, retinol binding protein and zinc in rheumatoid arthritis." *Clinical and Experimental Rheumatology.* 7 (1989): 465-69.

Kjeldsen-Kragh, Jens. "Dietary treatment of rheumatoid arthritis." *Scandinavian Journal of Rheumatology.* 63 (1996).

Kose, Kader et al. "Plasma selenium levels in rheumatoid arthritis." *Biological Trace Element Research.* 53 (1996): 51-56.

Krenner, J. M. et al. "Fish oil acid supplementation in active rheumatoid arthritis: A double-blinded, controlled, crossover study." *Annals of Internal Medicine* Vol. 106, no. 4 (1987): 497-503.

Latman, Neal S., and Robert Walls. "Personality and stress: An exploratory comparison of rheumatoid arthritis and osteoarthritis." *Archives of Physical Medicine and Rehabilitation.* 77 (1996): 796-800.

Murray, Michael T. *Natural Alternatives to Over-the-Counter and Prescription Drugs.* New York: William Morrow, 1994.

Rona, Zoltan P., and Jeanne Marie Martin. *Return to the Joy of Health.* Vancouver: Alive Books, 1995.

Skoldstam, L. "Fasting and vegan diet in rheumatoid arthritis." *Scandinavian Journal of Rheumatology.* Vol. 15, no. 2 (1987): 219-21.

Stammers, T. et al. "Fish oil in osteoarthritis." *Lancet.* 2 (1989): 503.

Zurier, Robert B. et al. "Gamma-linolenic acid treatment of rheumatoid arthritis: A randomized, placebo-controlled trial." *Arthritis and Rheumatism.* Vol. 39, no. 11 (1996): 1808-1817.

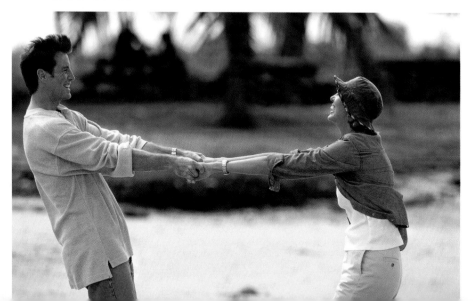

sources

To order an allergy testing kit contact:
York Nutritional Laboratory
Murton Way
Osbaldwick, York
United Kingdom
YO19 5US
Phone: +44 (0) 1904 410410
Fax: +44 (0) 1904 422000
E-mail: info@allergy.co.uk
http://www.allergy.co.uk/

Saliva testing:
One such lab offering this service is ZRT, located in
Beaverton, Oregon. You can reach them at:
Phone: (503) 466-2445
Fax: (503) 466-1636
E-mail: info@salivatest.com
http://www.salivatest.com

In addition to ZRT, the test is available through Great
Smokies Diagnostic Laboratory, but it only accepts tests
ordered by a doctor. Doctors can contact Great Smokies in
Asheville, North Carolina:
Phone: 1-800-522-4762
Fax: 1-828-285-9293
E-mail: cs@gsdl.com
http://www.gsdl.com
Costs vary between CAN $50 and $100 for each test.

The digestive enzyme Digeston, manufactured by Phytogenics,
is available from The Healing Arc http://www.thehealingarc.com

Platinum Naturals
Health Way Products
(A Division of Khang Health Products Ltd.)
11 Sims Cres., Units 4 & 5
Richmond Hill, Ontario L4B 1C9
Tel: (905) 731-8097
Toll Free: 1-800-668-5028
Fax: (905) 731-8116
Toll Free: 1-800-565-4586

Natren
310 S Willow Ln
West Lake Village, CA
91361 USA
Tel: (805) 371-4737 Ext. 110
Fax: (805) 371-4742

Natural Factors Nutritional Products Ltd.
3655 Bonneville Place,
Burnaby, BC, V3N 4S9
Tel: (604) 420-4229
Toll Free: 1-800-663-8900
Fax: (604) 420-0772
Toll Free- 1-800-663-2115

Remedies and supplements mentioned
in this book are available at quality
health food stores and nutrition centers.

First published in 2000 by
alive **books**
7436 Fraser Park Drive
Burnaby BC V5J 5B9
(604) 435–1919
1-800–661–0303

Book Design:
  Liza Novecoski
Artwork:
  Terence Yeung
  Raymond Cheung
Food Styling/Recipe Development:
  Fred Edrissi
Photography:
  Edmond Fong
  Siegfried Gursche
Photo Editing:
  Sabine Edrissi-Bredenbrock
Editing:
  Sandra Tonn
  Marian MacLean

Canadian Cataloguing in
Publication Data

Rona MD MSc, Zoltan
  Rheumatoid Arthritis

(*alive* natural health guides, 26
ISSN 1490-6503)
ISBN 1-55312-027-2

Printed in Canada

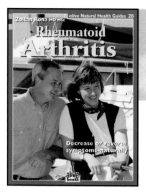

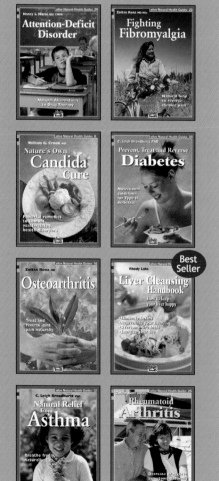
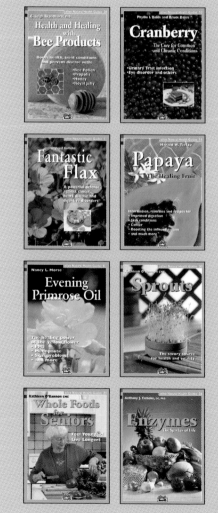